Starring: S

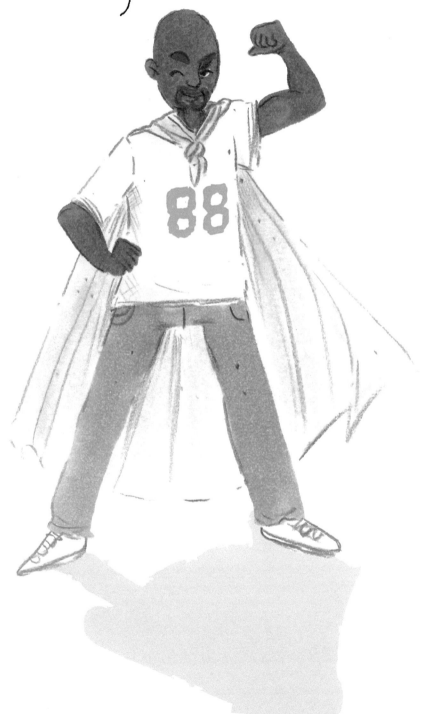

Printed in the United States of America

Butter Bird Books
www.ButterBirdBooks.com

ISBN-13: 978-1974190355
ISBN-10: 1974190358

Dedicated To "Pops"... "Dad"... "SUPERMAN"!
Even now I'm still learning to fly watching you

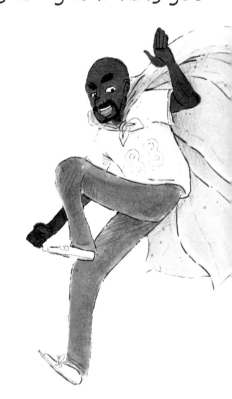

A Monster Named Cancer

Written by Moses A. Hardie III

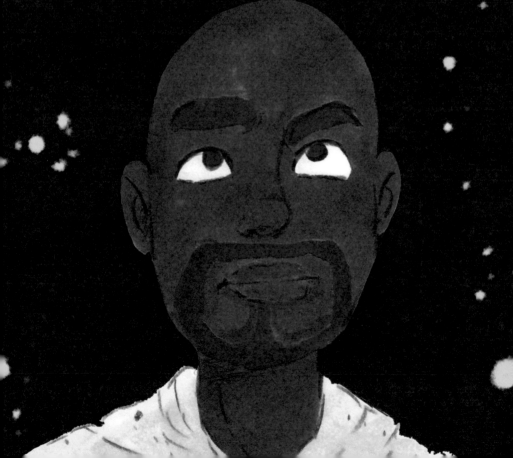

I'M LIL MOE

AND MY DADDY IS A   SUPER HERO!!!

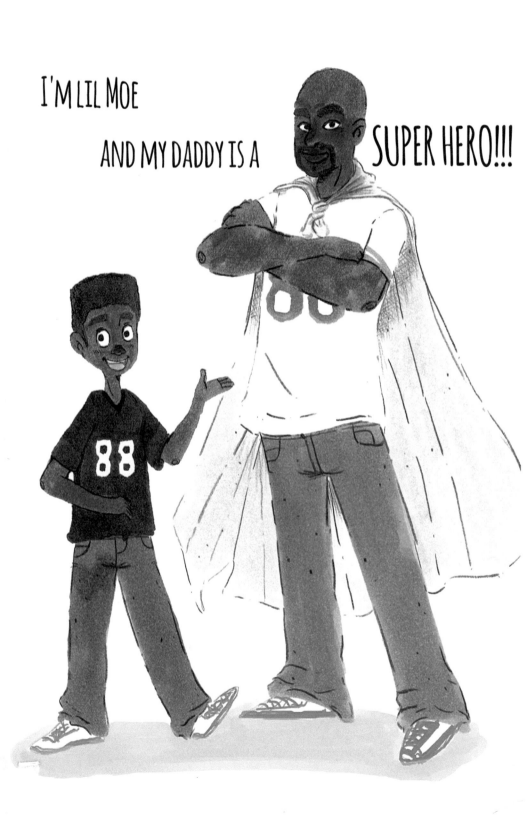

HE'S **STRONGER** THAN THE **STRONGEST GIANT**

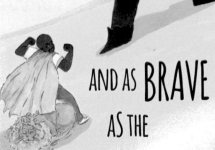

AND AS **BRAVE** AS THE **BRAVEST LION.**

HE COULD RUN EVEN **FASTER** THAN A SUPERSONIC JET

HI THERE MOON!

AND **JUMP** OVER THE MOON WITHOUT EVEN TRYIN'.

HE'S GOT MUSCLES ON TOP OF MUSCLES

AND CAN SEE **ALL** THE WAY INTO SPACE.

HE'S SMARTER THAN EVERY SCIENTIST, DOCTOR, AND TEACHER AND EVERYONE ELSE IN THE WHOLE HUMAN RACE.

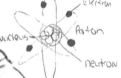

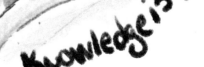

He's a kind and gentle man,
His heart is almost as big as the sun.

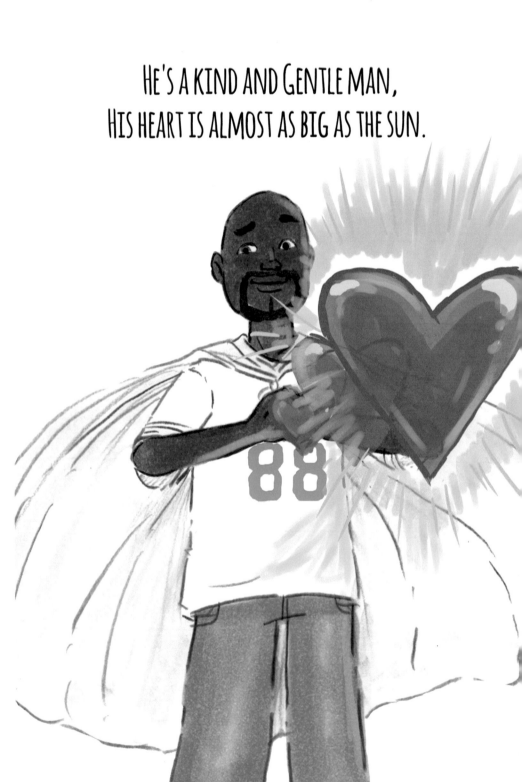

He works hard to make sure the family is safe, but he also knows how to have LOTS OF FUN!

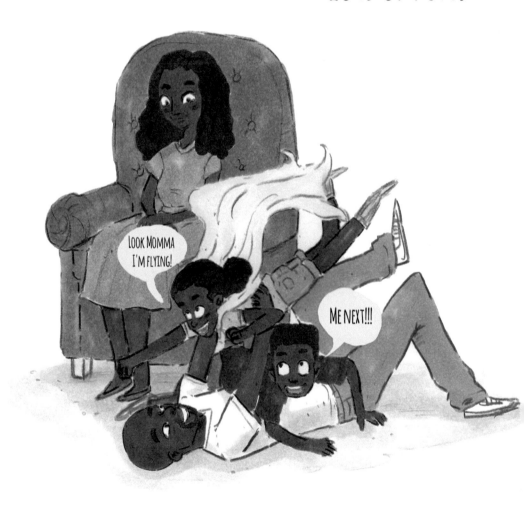

He's loved by many indeed,
      and tries to always do what is right.

And when there are bad guys that come around

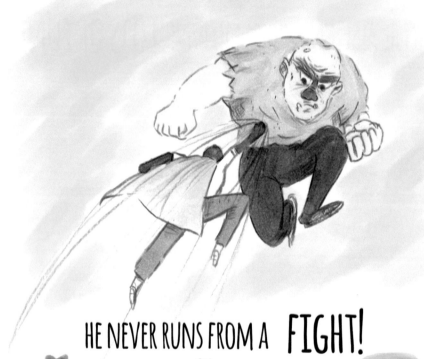

He never runs from a FIGHT!

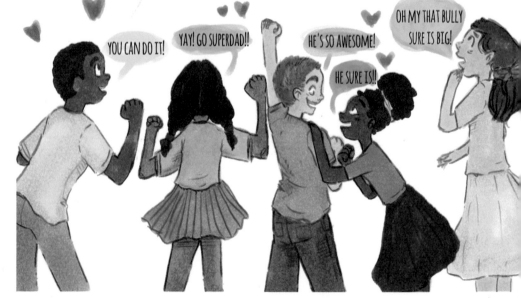

WELL THERE IS A NEW BAD GUY IN TOWN

AND HE WANTS TO TAKE ON SUPER DAD.

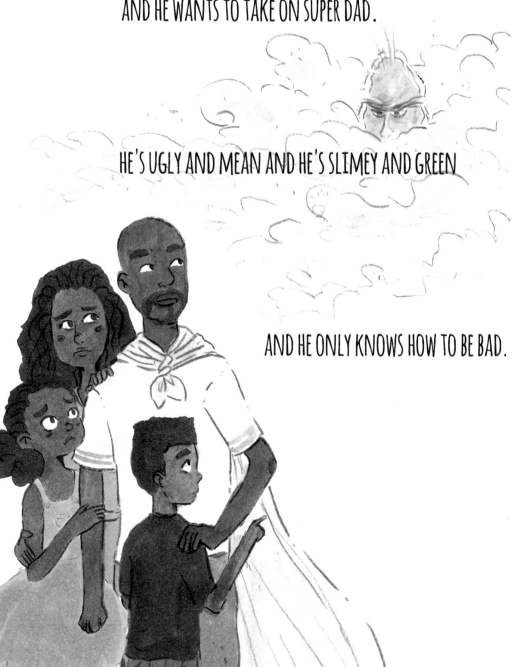

HE'S UGLY AND MEAN AND HE'S SLIMEY AND GREEN

AND HE ONLY KNOWS HOW TO BE BAD.

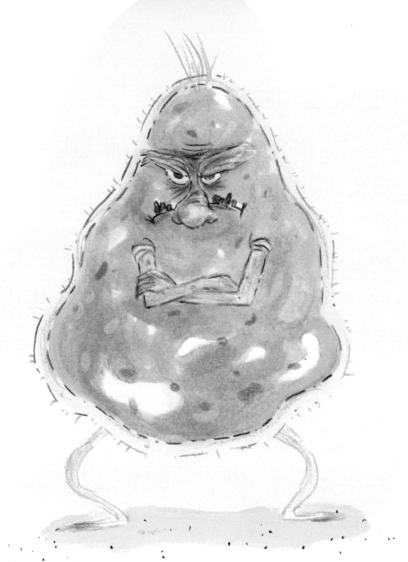

HE'S A **BIG** UGLY MONSTER NAMED CANCER.
HE'S GOT REDDISH EYES AND BROWN JAGGED TEETH.
HE HATES **EVERYONE** AND ONLY CAUSES PAIN,
AND HAS NO SOUL UNDERNEATH.

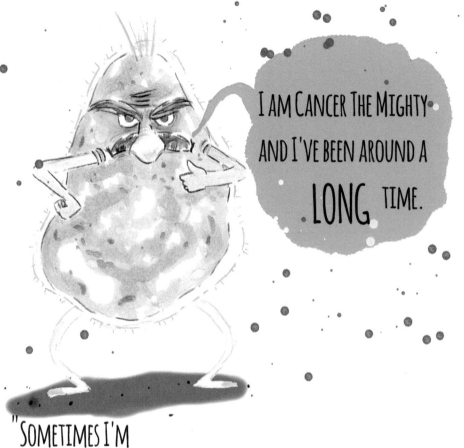

"Sometimes I'm LOUD AND YOU CAN HEAR ME COMING,

AND SOMETIMES I SNEAK UP WITHOUT A SIGN!"

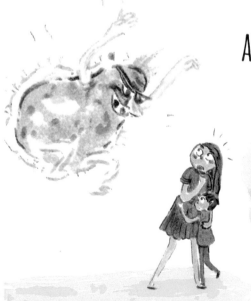

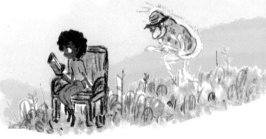

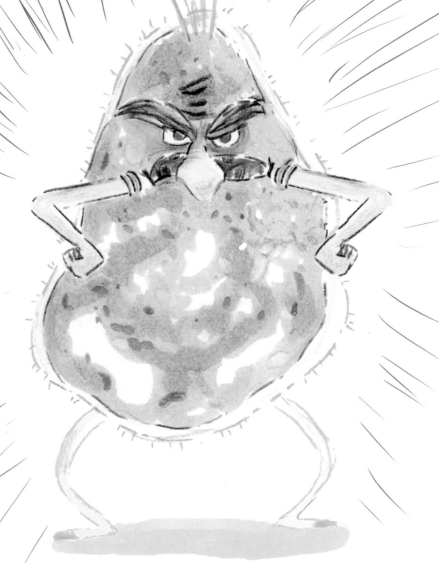

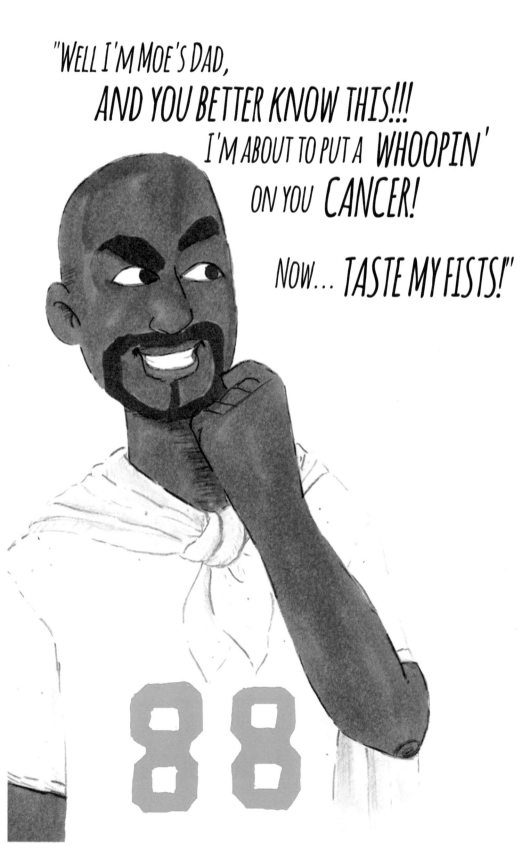

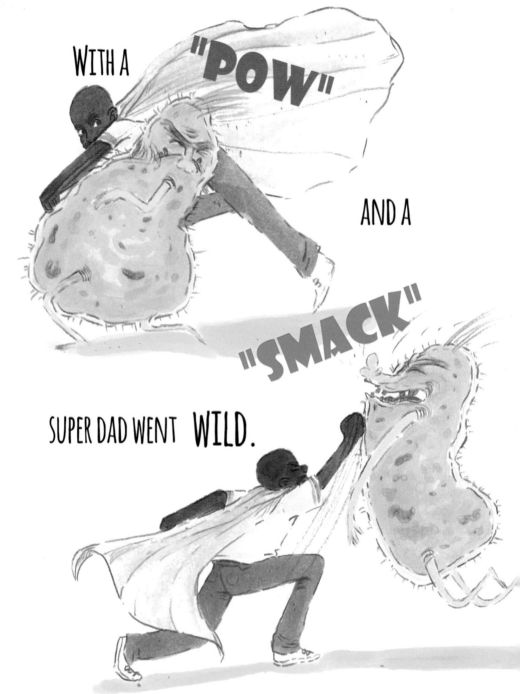

BUT THE CANCER MONSTER STOOD UP

AND HE STOOD UP QUICK AND FAST.

HE BRUSHED HIMSELF OFF

AND HE STARTED TO LAUGH.

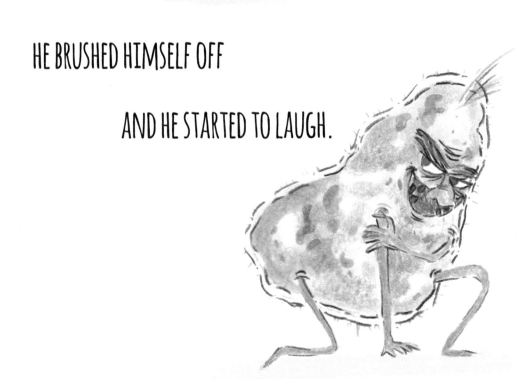

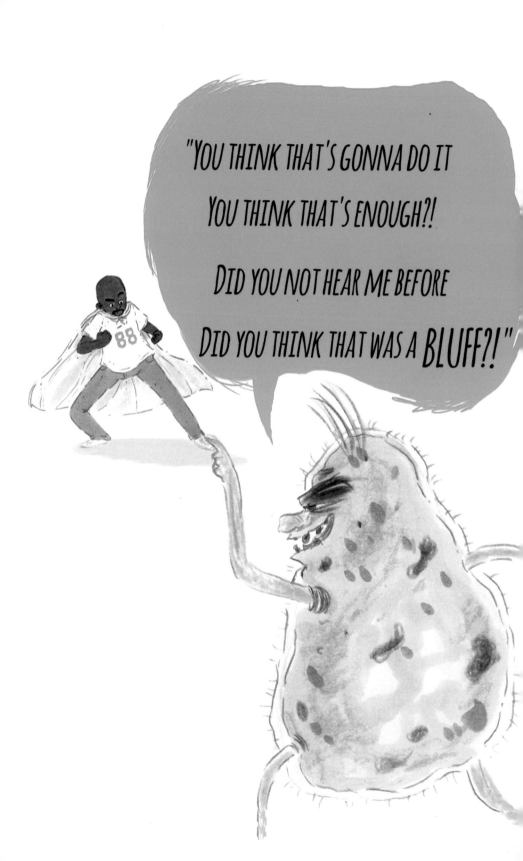

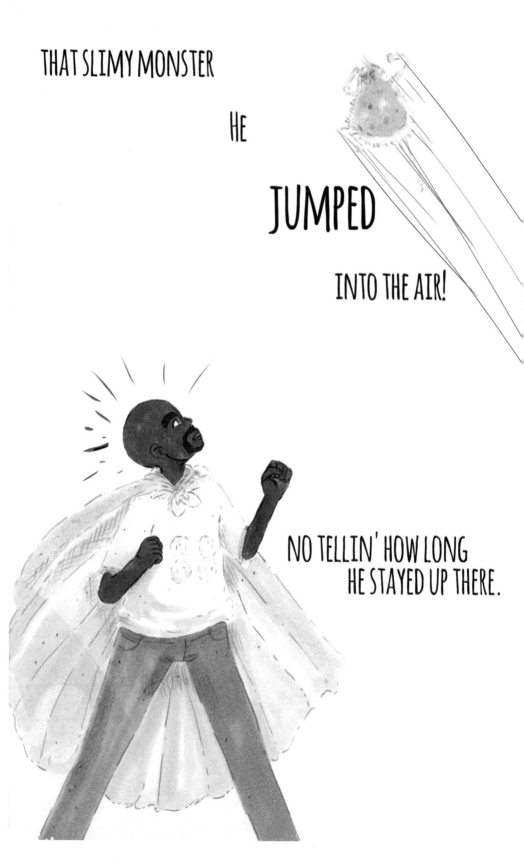

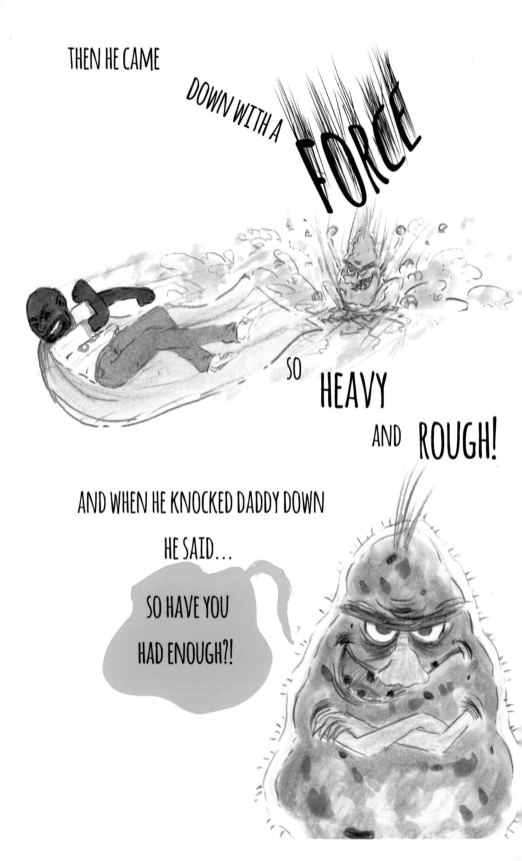

THEY FOUGHT AND THEY FOUGHT

IT SEEMED LIKE FOR MONTHS

BUT ONLY ONE WOULD WIN,

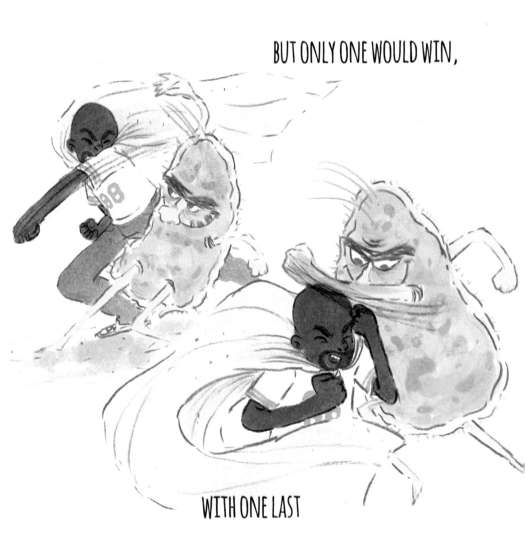

WITH ONE LAST

VICTORIOUS PUNCH!

AND WHEN THE SMOKE CLEARED
A FAMILIAR VOICE SAID...

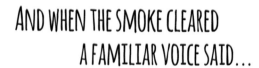

"IT'S OVER SON,
THE CANCER MONSTER IS
DEAD!"

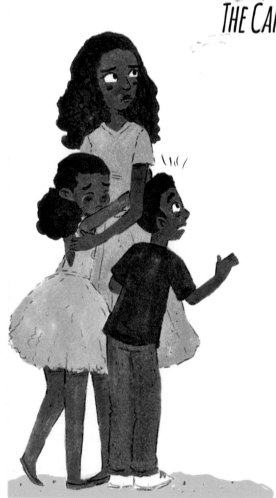

SO FOR THOSE STILL FIGHTING
STAND STRONG LIKE MY DAD.

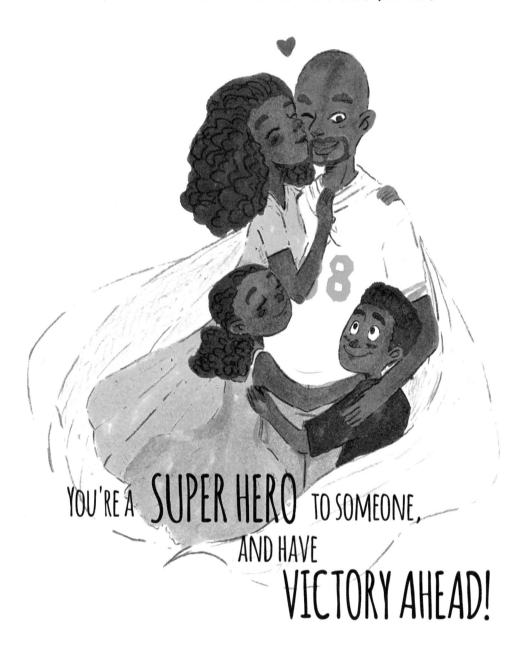

YOU'RE A **SUPER HERO** TO SOMEONE,
AND HAVE
VICTORY AHEAD!

Made in the USA
Columbia, SC
21 April 2024

34512838R00015